The Complete Gallbladder Health Guide

Prevention, Treatment, Post Surgery Care and Lifestyle for Recovery

Copyright © 2024

All rights reserved.

No part of this publication may be reproduced, distributed, or transmitted in any form or by any means, including photocopying, recording, or other electronic or mechanical methods, without the prior written permission of the author, except for the inclusion of brief quotations in a review or academic work, as permitted by copyright law.

Legal & Disclaimer:

The content provided in this book is for informational and educational purposes only. It is not intended to replace professional medical advice, diagnosis, or treatment. While all efforts have been made to ensure the accuracy and reliability of the information within, the author and publisher assume no responsibility for any errors or omissions. Readers are advised to consult a qualified healthcare provider before making any medical decisions, especially concerning gallbladder health, treatments, or post-surgery care.

The author and publisher are not responsible for any adverse effects, health issues, or complications arising from the use or application of information contained within this book. Each individual's health situation is unique, and medical advice should be tailored accordingly by a licensed professional.

The treatments, lifestyle recommendations, and dietary advice mentioned herein should not be considered a substitute for professional consultation. Any action taken by the reader is solely at their own risk.

Medical Disclaimer:

This book discusses medical topics related to gallbladder health, including prevention, treatment, and post-surgery care. It does not replace personalized medical guidance, and no claims are made regarding the effectiveness of treatments or remedies discussed. Always consult with a healthcare provider for advice tailored to your health circumstances.

Table of Contents

INTRODUCTION   **5**
ANATOMY AND FUNCTION OF THE GALLBLADDER   **8**
  Common Gallbladder Disorders   10
  Gallstones: Causes, Symptoms, and Diagnosis   13
    Formation of gallstones   13
    Symptoms of Gallstones Formation: Understanding the Prelude to Discomfort   16
    Cutting-Edge Technologies in Gallbladder Diagnosis and Treatment   19
  Cholecystitis: Inflammation of the Gallbladder   25
  The Role of Visceral Massage in Alleviating Gallbladder Pain   28
  Gallbladder Stones: A Time Bomb with Uncertain Outcomes   31
    Preserving or Removing the Gallbladder: A Matter of Consideration and Understanding   33
  Understanding Gallbladder Issues: A Holistic View from New German Medicine and Esoteric Insights   35
MANAGING GALLBLADDER ISSUES NATURALLY   **38**

Diet and Nutrition for Gallbladder Health	40
Starting Your Day Right: The Importance of a Balanced Breakfast	43
Lifestyle Changes to Support Gallbladder Function	45
Physical Exercise: A Cornerstone of Gallbladder Health	48
Herbal and Alternative Remedies	54
PART II: LIFE AFTER GALLBLADDER REMOVAL	**58**
Understanding Cholecystectomy: Surgery and Recovery	58
Post-Surgery Diet and Nutrition	61
CONCLUSION	**65**
LITERATURE	**68**
EXPLORE MORE GREAT READS	**75**

INTRODUCTION

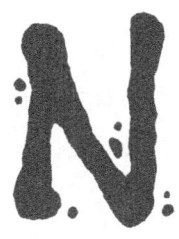

Navigating the complexities of gallbladder health extends beyond those who've undergone removal surgery; it's equally pertinent for individuals striving to preserve their gallbladder, aiming to alleviate pain, dissolve stones, and restore full functionality. As the author of this comprehensive guide, I've traversed the terrain of gallbladder health, dedicating over a year to understanding the spectrum of challenges faced by those striving to retain their gallbladder's health and those seeking guidance after surgical removal.

My personal quest for well-being sparked a deep dive into gallbladder health, spurred by firsthand experiences wrestling with discomfort, stone formation, and the uncertainties of surgical intervention. This book is an outcome of my quest for answers, amalgamating personal insights, medical expertise, and a fervent desire to extend a helping hand to individuals facing similar tribulations.

"The Complete Gallbladder Health Guide Prevention, Treatment, Post Surgery Care and Lifestyle for Recovery" isn't solely tailored for post-removal individuals; it's a comprehensive guide encompassing strategies for pain management, dietary considerations, and lifestyle adjustments for all stages of gallbladder health. Whether one seeks to preserve their gallbladder, dissolve stones, regain functionality, or adjust to life post-surgery, the recipes and guidance within these pages serve as a compass.

Through meticulous research and consultations, this guide articulates the significance of diet, stress management, and holistic approaches for gallbladder well-being. It doesn't just offer recipes; it presents a spectrum of solutions-practical, dietary, and emotional—for those embarking on a journey toward gallbladder health and those embracing life after its removal.

This book stands as a beacon of hope for anyone seeking relief, empowerment, and a renewed perspective on gallbladder health. It's my fervent aspiration that this guide becomes a companion, offering solace, empowerment, and a roadmap toward living well despite the challenges of gallbladder-related concerns.

Anatomy and Function of the Gallbladder

The gallbladder, a seemingly unassuming organ tucked beneath the liver, plays a pivotal role in our digestive system. Often overlooked until trouble arises, this small, pear-shaped pouch acts as a reservoir for bile, the golden elixir crucial for fat digestion and absorption.

Picture this: nestled snugly against the underside of the liver, the gallbladder resembles a miniature pouch, about 7-10 centimeters in length when fully distended.

Its primary function? To store and concentrate bile, that unsung hero produced by the liver cells, which journeys through intricate bile ducts to reach its destination.

Bile, often likened to a digestive detergent, is a concoction of bile salts, cholesterol, bilirubin, and other compounds essential for breaking down dietary fats. Here's where the gallbladder steps in, acting as a storage facility for this vital fluid. When we consume a meal, especially one rich in fats, the gallbladder contracts, releasing concentrated bile into the small intestine through the bile ducts.

This release of bile facilitates the emulsification of fats, breaking them down into smaller droplets that enzymes find easier to digest. Imagine the gallbladder as a strategic partner in the digestive orchestra, precisely timing the release of bile to ensure efficient fat breakdown, absorption of vital nutrients, and the body's energy supply.

However, this seemingly humble organ isn't without its woes. Gallstones, those crystalline formations composed of cholesterol or bilirubin, can form within the gallbladder, leading to discomfort, pain, and even inflammation. Such conditions can disrupt the gallbladder's function, impacting its ability to store and release bile effectively, and sometimes necessitating its removal.

Understanding the gallbladder's anatomy and function underscores the significance of its role in our digestive symphony. It serves as a reminder of the intricate mechanisms orchestrating our body's digestion, urging us to nurture and care for this often-forgotten yet indispensable organ. From dietary choices to lifestyle habits, preserving gallbladder health becomes a cornerstone in fostering overall well-being and digestive harmony.

Common Gallbladder Disorders

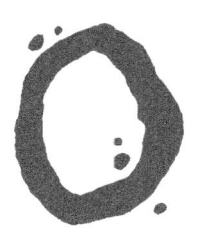

One prevalent issue affecting the gallbladder is the formation of gallstones. These crystalline formations, often composed of cholesterol or bilirubin, can range in size from minuscule specks to substantial stones that impede the gallbladder's function. These stones may not elicit symptoms initially, but they can lead to excruciating pain if they obstruct the bile ducts, causing what is commonly known as a gallbladder «attack.» These attacks manifest as intense upper abdominal pain, often radiating to the back or shoulder, accompanied by nausea and vomiting.

Cholecystitis, another common disorder, involves inflammation of the gallbladder. This inflammation can be acute or chronic, with acute cases typically stemming from gallstones obstructing the cystic duct, leading to a buildup of bile and subsequent inflammation. Chronic cholecystitis may develop over time, marked by repeated bouts of inflammation that gradually impair the gallbladder's function.

Gallbladder polyps, though less common, are growths that can develop within the gallbladder wall. While most polyps are benign, some have the potential to become cancerous. Monitoring these polyps through imaging studies and, in some cases, surgical removal might be necessary to prevent complications.

Biliary dyskinesia, characterized by abnormal gallbladder contractions, can result in inefficient bile release, causing symptoms akin to those of gallstones or cholecystitis. Patients may experience abdominal pain and digestive disturbances without the presence of gallstones.

The diagnosis of gallbladder disorders often involves a combination of medical history assessment, physical examination, and imaging tests like ultrasound or CT scans. Treatment strategies vary depending on the specific disorder and its severity. Gallstones may be managed through medication to dissolve them, but surgical removal of the gallbladder, known as cholecystectomy, is a common and effective solution, often relieving symptoms and preventing recurrence.

Lifestyle modifications play a pivotal role in managing and preventing gallbladder disorders. A balanced diet, low in saturated fats and cholesterol, can reduce the risk of gallstone formation. Incorporating fiber-rich foods, staying hydrated, and avoiding rapid weight fluctuations contribute to overall gallbladder health.

In conclusion, understanding the spectrum of common gallbladder disorders empowers individuals to recognize symptoms, seek timely medical intervention, and adopt preventive measures. These insights underscore the importance of digestive health and highlight the significance of nurturing habits conducive to gallbladder well-being, ultimately fostering a harmonious relationship with this often-underestimated yet vital organ.

Gallstones: Causes, Symptoms, and Diagnosis

Formation of gallstones

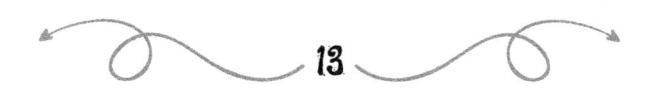

The formation of gallstones, a fascinating yet potentially troublesome occurrence within the gallbladder, unveils a complex interplay of biological factors. These crystalline formations, often composed of cholesterol or bilirubin, represent a significant concern in digestive health, warranting a deeper exploration into their intricate genesis.

At the core of gallstone formation lies an imbalance in the constituents of bile, the golden elixir produced by the liver to aid in fat digestion. When this delicate equilibrium is disrupted, it sets the stage for the genesis of these crystalline structures. Cholesterol gallstones, the most prevalent type, typically stem from an excess of cholesterol in bile. This surplus cholesterol precipitates into solid crystals, gradually forming into stones within the gallbladder.

The cascade of events leading to cholesterol gallstone formation is multifaceted. It often begins with the supersaturation of bile with cholesterol, where the cholesterol concentration surpasses the fluid's capacity to dissolve it. Under such conditions, cholesterol starts to crystallize, forming microscopic particles known as microcrystals. These minute particles, akin to a seed, serve as the nucleus for gallstone development.

However, the journey from microcrystals to substantial gallstones isn't immediate. These nascent crystals require time and conditions conducive to their growth and aggregation. Factors such as stasis or reduced motility within the gallbladder, which impedes the complete emptying of bile, create an environment ripe for these microcrystals to conglomerate. Over time, these aggregations of cholesterol crystals merge and solidify, evolving into the palpable gallstones that can vary in size and composition.

Pigment gallstones, less common than their cholesterol counterparts, form through a different mechanism. These stones result from an excess of bilirubin, a breakdown product of red blood cells, which accumulates in bile. High levels of bilirubin can lead to the precipitation and aggregation of bilirubin molecules, resulting in the formation of pigment stones.

The journey through gallstone formation can be silent, with these crystalline structures residing within the gallbladder without causing noticeable symptoms. However, when these stones obstruct the flow of bile or trigger spasms within the gallbladder, they can elicit a range of uncomfortable sensations, including acute and intense pain in the abdomen, often radiating to the back or shoulder.

In essence, the genesis of gallstones is a complex amalgamation of cholesterol or bilirubin imbalance, supersaturation of bile, and conducive conditions within the gallbladder.

Understanding this intricate process underscores the importance of maintaining bile equilibrium and adopting habits conducive to gallbladder health. This comprehension serves as a cornerstone in proactive management, ultimately fostering digestive harmony and well-being.

Symptoms of Gallstones Formation: Understanding the Prelude to Discomfort

The formation of gallstones within the gallbladder, while often asymptomatic in its early stages, can gradually manifest into a range of discomforting sensations and symptoms. Delving into the nuanced landscape of these symptoms provides a crucial insight into the evolving narrative of gallstone formation and its impact on an individual's well-being.

At the inception of gallstone formation, individuals might not experience any overt symptoms. These crystalline formations can exist silently within the gallbladder, gradually developing without causing noticeable discomfort. However, as these stones grow in size or migrate within the gallbladder, they can provoke a cascade of sensations, signaling the body's response to their presence.

One of the hallmark symptoms attributed to gallstone formation is biliary colic—an abrupt onset of intense, gripping pain in the upper abdomen or right shoulder. This pain, often described as excruciating and intermittent, can persist for hours and typically occurs after consuming fatty or heavy meals. The severity of this pain can disrupt daily activities, leading individuals to seek immediate medical attention.

Accompanying this intense pain, individuals might experience nausea and vomiting. These symptoms often arise as a consequence of the gallstones obstructing the bile ducts or triggering spasms within the gallbladder. The distress caused by these symptoms can significantly impact an individual's quality of life, leading to discomfort, anxiety, and a decreased appetite.

In some cases, particularly when gallstones cause inflammation of the gallbladder (cholecystitis), additional symptoms might emerge. These can include fever, persistent abdominal pain that doesn't subside, and tenderness in the abdomen upon touch, signaling a more acute phase in the progression of gallstone-related complications.

Notably, while some individuals might experience pronounced symptoms indicative of gallstone formation, others may remain asymptomatic, unaware of the presence of these crystalline entities until detected incidentally during routine medical examinations or imaging studies.

Accurate diagnosis of gallstones and their associated symptoms often involves a comprehensive evaluation by healthcare professionals. Imaging techniques like ultrasound, CT scans, or MRIs play a pivotal role in visualizing gallstones within the gallbladder and determining their size, quantity, and potential impact on an individual's health.

In essence, understanding the nuanced symptoms associated with gallstone formation is pivotal in recognizing potential issues and seeking timely medical intervention. These symptoms, often characterized by intense abdominal pain, nausea, and vomiting, serve as red flags prompting individuals to navigate towards proactive management and preventive measures conducive to gallbladder health.

Cutting-Edge Technologies in Gallbladder Diagnosis and Treatment

As medical science advances at an unprecedented pace, new technologies are revolutionizing the way we approach gallbladder health. These innovations not only enhance our ability to diagnose issues with greater precision but also offer less invasive treatment options, promising improved outcomes and faster recovery times for patients grappling with gallbladder disorders.

Advanced Imaging Techniques:

1. **High-Resolution Ultrasound:** Gone are the days of grainy, difficult-to-interpret ultrasound images. Modern high-resolution ultrasound technology provides crystal-clear visualizations of the gallbladder and surrounding structures. This leap in imaging quality allows for the detection of even the tiniest gallstones, some as small as 1-2 millimeters, which might have been missed by conventional ultrasound. Moreover, advanced Doppler capabilities enable real-time assessment of blood flow, aiding in the diagnosis of inflammatory conditions like acute cholecystitis.

2. **Magnetic Resonance Cholangiopancreatography (MRCP):** This non-invasive imaging technique uses powerful magnetic fields and radio waves to create detailed images of the biliary and pancreatic ducts. MRCP excels in detecting obstructions, strictures, and even subtle anatomical variations that might contribute to gallbladder issues. Unlike traditional

cholangiography, MRCP doesn't require the injection of contrast material, making it safer and more comfortable for patients.

3. **Endoscopic Ultrasound (EUS):** Combining the precision of endoscopy with the non-invasive nature of ultrasound, EUS offers unparalleled imaging of the gallbladder and biliary system. A thin, flexible tube with an ultrasound probe at its tip is inserted through the mouth and into the upper digestive tract. This proximity allows for high-resolution imaging and can even guide fine-needle aspiration for tissue sampling when necessary.

Innovative Treatment Modalities:

1. **Robotic-Assisted Cholecystectomy:** While laparoscopic cholecystectomy has been the gold standard for gallbladder removal, robotic-assisted surgery takes precision to the next level. Using a sophisticated robotic system, surgeons can perform intricate movements with enhanced dexterity and 3D visualization. This technology allows for smaller incisions,

reduced postoperative pain, and potentially faster recovery times.

2. **Single-Incision Laparoscopic Surgery (SILS):** For those concerned about cosmetic outcomes, SILS offers a nearly scarless approach to gallbladder removal. By making a single incision through the navel, surgeons can remove the gallbladder without leaving visible scars on the abdomen. While technically challenging, this approach is gaining popularity for its excellent cosmetic results and potentially reduced postoperative pain.

3. **Gallstone Dissolution Techniques:** For patients who are poor surgical candidates or prefer non-surgical options, new gallstone dissolution techniques offer hope. Advanced oral medications that dissolve cholesterol-based gallstones are under development, promising a non-invasive alternative to surgery for select patients.

4. **Lithotripsy Advancements:** While shock wave lithotripsy for gallstones isn't new, recent advancements

have improved its efficacy and safety profile. Newer lithotripters use more focused energy waves, reducing damage to surrounding tissues while more effectively fragmenting gallstones.

5. **Cholecystoscopy:** This minimally invasive procedure allows direct visualization of the gallbladder's interior using a thin, flexible scope. It's particularly useful for diagnosing and treating conditions like gallbladder polyps or investigating unexplained biliary pain when other imaging studies are inconclusive.

The Promise of Artificial Intelligence:

The integration of artificial intelligence (AI) in gallbladder health management is perhaps one of the most exciting frontiers. AI algorithms are being developed to:

- Analyze ultrasound images with greater accuracy, potentially detecting gallstones and other abnormalities that might be missed by human eyes.

- Predict the likelihood of gallstone formation based

on patient data, allowing for more targeted preventive strategies.

- Optimize surgical planning for complex cases, helping surgeons choose the most appropriate approach for each individual patient.

While many of these technologies are still in various stages of development and implementation, they represent the cutting edge of gallbladder care. As with any medical advancement, it's crucial to approach these innovations with both excitement and caution. The long-term effects and outcomes of some of these technologies are still being studied.

As we embrace these technological advancements, it's important to remember that they complement, rather than replace, the fundamental principles of gallbladder health we've discussed throughout this book. A balanced diet, regular exercise, and attentiveness to your body's signals remain the cornerstones of maintaining a healthy gallbladder.

In the rapidly evolving landscape of medical technology, staying informed and engaged with your healthcare provider is key. They can help you understand which of these new technologies might be most beneficial for your specific situation, ensuring you receive the most appropriate and effective care for your gallbladder health.

Cholecystitis: Inflammation of the Gallbladder

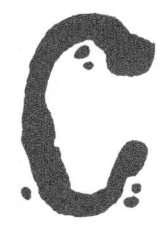

Cholecystitis, an inflammation of the gallbladder, presents a tumultuous chapter in the narrative of digestive health. This condition, often arising from gallstones obstructing the cystic duct, marks a significant departure from the silent existence of these crystalline formations, catapulting individuals into a realm of discomfort and potential complications.

At its core, cholecystitis is a consequence of obstructed bile flow within the gallbladder. Gallstones, those crystalline entities formed from cholesterol or bilirubin, can hinder the proper drainage of bile, leading to a buildup of this digestive fluid within the gallbladder. This stagnant bile serves as a breeding ground for inflammation, initiating a cascade of events that result in gallbladder irritation, swelling, and pain.

The hallmark of cholecystitis is persistent and intense abdominal pain, typically localized in the upper right quadrant. This pain, distinct from the intermittent biliary colic associated with gallstone formation, often lingers for hours or days, becoming more relentless and debilitating. It might radiate to the right shoulder or back and intensify after consuming fatty or greasy foods. Accompanying this pain, individuals might experience tenderness in the abdomen upon touch, further exacerbating their discomfort.

As cholecystitis progresses, additional symptoms may manifest, signaling a more acute phase of gallbladder inflammation. Fever, chills, and an elevated white blood cell count might indicate the body's heightened immune response to the inflamed gallbladder, suggesting a potential infection complicating the condition.

Diagnosing cholecystitis involves a thorough medical evaluation, including a review of symptoms, physical examination, and imaging studies. Ultrasound imaging remains a primary diagnostic tool, allowing visualization of gallbladder inflammation, thickened gallbladder walls, and the presence of gallstones or related complications.

Management of cholecystitis often necessitates medical intervention, especially in severe or recurrent cases. In acute cholecystitis, treatment might involve fasting to rest the gallbladder, intravenous fluids for hydration, and antibiotics to address any associated infection. Surgical removal of the gallbladder, known as cholecystectomy, is often considered the definitive solution, offering relief from recurrent inflammation and preventing future complications.

Prevention of cholecystitis revolves around mitigating gallstone formation and adopting lifestyle changes conducive to gallbladder health. This includes maintaining a balanced diet, avoiding rapid weight fluctuations, and steering clear of excessive consumption of high-fat or greasy foods.

In essence, understanding cholecystitis and its associated symptoms is pivotal in navigating potential complications arising from gallstone-related inflammation. This comprehension underscores the importance of timely medical intervention, proactive management, and preventive measures aimed at preserving gallbladder health and fostering digestive harmony.

The Role of Visceral Massage in Alleviating Gallbladder Pain

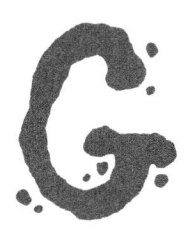

Gallbladder attacks are notorious for their excruciating pain and discomfort, often prompting a quest for immediate relief. In this pursuit, visceral massage emerges as a promising therapeutic intervention, offering potential comfort and relief during these distressing episodes.

Visceral massage, a specialized technique targeting internal organs, aims to release tension, enhance circulation, and restore optimal function within the body. Specifically tailored for the abdomen, this technique involves gentle, rhythmic manipulation designed to alleviate tension and induce relaxation.

During a gallbladder attack, the intensity of pain stemming from gallstones or inflammation can be overwhelming. Visceral massage, skillfully administered by a trained practitioner, focuses on the affected abdominal area. By applying gentle pressure and specific massage techniques, it seeks to reduce tension, potentially providing relief amidst the acute discomfort of an attack.

The mechanics of visceral massage are rooted in its ability to stimulate the parasympathetic nervous system, promoting a state of relaxation. This relaxation response can potentially alleviate spasms, ease constriction within bile ducts, and offer respite from the sharp, stabbing pain characteristic of gallbladder attacks.

Beyond immediate pain relief, regular sessions of visceral massage may contribute to overall gallbladder health. By improving circulation, reducing tension in the abdominal region, and optimizing organ function, it may play a role in preventing or reducing the frequency of gallbladder-related issues.

However, it's important to regard visceral massage as a supplementary, rather than sole, therapeutic approach for gallbladder problems. When integrated with conventional medical treatments, it can offer additional support and relief. Consulting healthcare professionals is paramount before considering visceral massage, especially in cases of acute or severe symptoms. Their assessment ensures the massage is safe, appropriate, and beneficial for individual circumstances.

In conclusion, visceral massage stands as a non-invasive and potentially effective method for managing the intense pain accompanying gallbladder attacks. Its emphasis on inducing relaxation and reducing tension within the abdominal area presents a complementary approach to conventional treatments. When administered by a qualified professional and in conjunction with medical advice, visceral massage holds promise as a tool to mitigate the severity of gallbladder-related pain and discomfort.

Gallbladder Stones: A Time Bomb with Uncertain Outcomes

The presence of gallbladder stones is akin to a ticking time bomb, the detonation of which remains unpredictable, carrying unforeseen consequences for an individual's health and well-being. The uncertainty surrounding when and how these stones might cause distress looms ominously.

Gallbladder stones, often silent in their formation, can escalate into severe complications at any moment. The intermittent nature of symptoms, ranging from mild discomfort to excruciating pain, renders the situation precarious. The unpredictability of a stone's movement within the bile ducts brings forth the looming threat of acute episodes, leading to severe pain, jaundice, or even pancreatitis.

Furthermore, an untreated gallbladder with stones can adversely affect the functioning of other vital organs, primarily the liver and pancreas. The gallbladder's role in storing and releasing bile, essential for fat digestion, can be disrupted. The imbalance in bile flow not only affects digestion but also exerts undue stress on the liver and pancreas. Over time, this stress may contribute to liver issues or pancreatitis, amplifying the complexities of the situation.

The intricate relationship between the gallbladder, liver, and pancreas underscores the interdependency of these organs in the digestive process. An ailing gallbladder not only jeopardizes its own functionality but also disrupts the harmonious coordination among these vital organs, potentially triggering a cascade of health issues.

Neglecting the removal of a gallbladder plagued by stones is akin to playing a hazardous waiting game. The risks associated with such a gamble extend beyond the occasional discomfort to the realm of severe complications and long-term organ dysfunction. Consequently, the decision to delay intervention can exacerbate the situation, posing a significant threat to an individual's health and overall well-being.

In conclusion, the presence of gallbladder stones should not be taken lightly. It's imperative to recognize their potential to wreak havoc on the body, not only through acute episodes but also through long-term repercussions on essential organs. Timely intervention and the removal of the gallbladder, when necessary, stand as critical measures to prevent the ticking time bomb of gallstones from causing irreparable harm.

Preserving or Removing the Gallbladder: A Matter of Consideration and Understanding

The decision to retain or remove the gallbladder hinges on specific circumstances and the patient's condition. However, there are situations where fear of surgery and misunderstanding of risks might lead to choosing to retain the gallbladder, which in some cases could heighten health risks.

Many individuals fear surgeries and opt to keep their gallbladder, even when it becomes problematic. They might consult doctors offering methods to dissolve stones, hoping to avoid surgery. However, this approach might be temporary and fails to address the underlying cause of stone formation. Moreover, even if stones are fragmented, they can recur, causing further episodes.

In cases of gallstone formation and ignoring symptoms, there's a risk of bile duct blockage. When stones move, they can cause severe pain, but attempting to maneuver them through the body can result in a risk of fatality. In such instances, surgery may become the sole means to prevent severe complications.

Furthermore, the gallbladder should not be retained if it's non-functional, doesn't contract, is completely obstructed by stones, and fails to perform its function.

Understanding the risks and potential complications of

keeping a problematic gallbladder is crucial. Surgery, contrary to popular belief, is often minimally invasive, and individuals recover quickly, leading pain-free lives. The fear of surgery shouldn't outweigh the potential health hazards associated with retaining a dysfunctional gallbladder.

Understanding Gallbladder Issues: A Holistic View from New German Medicine and Esoteric Insights

In the realm of holistic healing, the connection between emotional well-being and physical health stands as a fundamental tenet. According to the principles of New German Medicine and esoteric perspectives, issues concerning the gallbladder often intertwine with an individual's emotional landscape and energy dynamics.

The core thesis posits that emotional states, particularly negative ones like anger and aggression, can significantly impact the health of the gallbladder. When a person navigates a lifestyle or circumstances where they feel compelled to defend their territory or personal space, these emotions can manifest and create disturbances within the gallbladder's functioning. It is believed that these emotions can lead to stagnation or uncontrolled releases of bile, ultimately contributing to the formation of gallstones and subsequent issues.

Living in a state of chronic stress, perpetually without relaxation or moments of mental calmness, also contributes to this scenario. Stress amplifies the negative emotional responses and exacerbates the potential for disruptions in the gallbladder's equilibrium.

The intricate connection between emotions and physical health, particularly regarding the gallbladder, underscores the importance of addressing emotional well-being in holistic treatment approaches. Techniques such as meditation and relaxation practices play a pivotal role in rebalancing emotional states and reducing stress. By fostering a sense of mental tranquility and releasing pent-up negative emotions, individuals can potentially alleviate the burden on the gallbladder and mitigate the risk of issues associated with bile stasis and stone formation.

In the context of gallbladder treatment, it's crucial to consider this holistic perspective. Beyond conventional medical interventions, integrating practices that promote emotional balance, stress reduction, and relaxation into the treatment regimen could offer comprehensive care and potentially prevent recurrence of gallbladder issues.

In conclusion, New German Medicine and esoteric viewpoints emphasize the intricate interplay between emotions, stress, and gallbladder health. Acknowledging and addressing emotional well-being, incorporating relaxation practices, and fostering mental equilibrium stand as vital components in holistic approaches to gallbladder health and healing. Integrating these holistic practices alongside conventional medical treatments could pave the way for a more comprehensive and effective approach to managing gallbladder issues.

Managing Gallbladder Issues Naturally

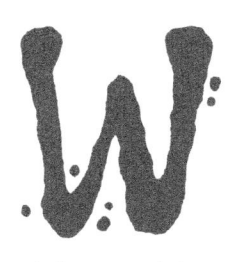

When it comes to treating gallbladder issues using herbs and natural remedies, it's crucial to realize that self-treatment without consulting a doctor can be both risky and inappropriate. If an individual chooses to use herbs or natural methods to eliminate gallstones, they should be under the supervision of a qualified medical professional.

Self-medication can lead to serious complications, especially concerning gallstones. Uncontrolled use of herbs or unprofessional therapy may cause the movement or blockage of gallstones, or even their fragmentation, leading to acute pain and severe complications.

It's important to note that even when using herbs or natural methods, regular monitoring of gallstone status through ultrasound examinations (ultrasounds) under a doctor's supervision is essential. This allows tracking the effectiveness of the chosen therapy and preventing potential complications associated with self-treatment.

Decisions regarding treating gallbladder issues with herbs or natural remedies should be made in consultation with a medical professional. They can evaluate the patient's condition, assess potential risks, and choose the most effective and safe treatment.

Diet and Nutrition for Gallbladder Health

The gallbladder, a small yet integral part of the digestive system, plays a crucial role in storing and concentrating bile—a fluid that aids in digesting fats. Problems related to bile flow and discomfort in the gallbladder often call for dietary adjustments aimed at easing symptoms and promoting better digestive health.

Understanding the Role of Diet in Gallbladder Health:

Diet plays a pivotal role in managing conditions associated with bile flow issues and gallbladder discomfort. Certain dietary choices can either alleviate or exacerbate symptoms, emphasizing the importance of a well-balanced and mindful eating regimen.

Foods to Avoid:

Fatty, greasy, and fried foods are commonly recognized

as triggers for gallbladder discomfort. These foods stimulate the gallbladder to release bile, potentially causing pain or discomfort, especially in those prone to gallbladder issues. Additionally, highly processed foods, refined sugars, and excessive consumption of red meat may contribute to exacerbating symptoms.

Gallbladder-Friendly Foods:

In contrast, incorporating a diet rich in fiber, fresh fruits, vegetables, and lean proteins can support gallbladder health. Fiber aids in digestion and helps regulate cholesterol levels, potentially reducing the risk of gallstone formation. Foods high in omega-3 fatty acids, such as salmon or flaxseeds, may have anti-inflammatory properties, potentially benefiting individuals experiencing gallbladder discomfort.

Hydration and Moderation:

Staying adequately hydrated is crucial for maintaining gallbladder health. Drinking sufficient water throughout the day can aid in the digestion and flow of bile, potentially reducing the risk of gallstone formation. Moreover, portion control and moderation in meal sizes can prevent overwhelming the gallbladder with excessive amounts of food at once, reducing the chances of discomfort.

Meal Timing and Consistency:

Establishing regular meal times and avoiding prolonged fasting can help maintain consistent bile flow. Skipping meals or prolonged periods without eating might cause the gallbladder to contract less frequently, potentially leading to stagnant bile and discomfort.

Conclusion:

In essence, adopting a gallbladder-friendly diet involves making thoughtful food choices that support digestive health. Prioritizing whole foods, fiber-rich options, lean proteins, staying hydrated, and maintaining portion control can contribute significantly to managing symptoms related to bile flow issues and gallbladder discomfort. However, individual responses to dietary changes may vary, so consulting a healthcare professional or a registered dietitian is advisable for personalized guidance in managing gallbladder-related concerns through dietary modifications.

Starting Your Day Right: The Importance of a Balanced Breakfast

Beginning your day with a well-rounded breakfast sets the tone for your body's functions and energy levels. It's not about overindulgence or consuming high-fat meals but rather about incorporating essential elements like fats, omega-3s, and vegetables in moderate amounts.

The Balanced Breakfast Formula:

A balanced breakfast should ideally include a moderate amount of fats, particularly those containing omega-3 fatty acids, alongside vegetables. This isn't about excessive fats but rather a healthy dose sufficient for facilitating bile flow and kickstarting the digestive system.

Focusing on Healthy Fats and Omega-3s:

Incorporating sources of healthy fats and omega-3s, such as avocados, nuts, or seeds, in your breakfast can support gallbladder health and aid in digestion. These fats, in controlled portions, play a vital role in promoting bile flow without overwhelming the system.

The Role of Bitter and Acidic Foods:

Including bitter and acidic foods in your breakfast can also contribute to stimulating bile flow. Some types of greens, known for their bitter taste, and fermented or pickled vegetables with their acidic nature can trigger the release of bile, aiding in the digestive process.

A Balanced Approach:

It's crucial to strike a balance; the objective isn't to load up on excessive fats or heavy foods but to incorporate a variety of elements that support digestion and gallbladder health. Small amounts of the right fats, omega-3 sources, and a mix of vegetables, bitter greens, and acidic foods can initiate bile flow without causing discomfort.

Conclusion:

Starting your day with a breakfast that includes these elements in moderation sets the stage for a well-functioning digestive system. It's about providing your body with the right components to kickstart digestion and ensure gallbladder health, without overloading your system. This balanced approach to breakfast can promote optimal digestion and overall well-being throughout the day.

Lifestyle Changes to Support Gallbladder Function

Beyond dietary adjustments, lifestyle changes play a pivotal role in supporting gallbladder health and preventing potential discomfort or complications. Embracing certain habits and modifications in daily routines can significantly contribute to the well-being of this crucial digestive organ.

Hydration and Fluid Intake:

Maintaining adequate hydration is fundamental for gallbladder health. Drinking sufficient water throughout the day facilitates bile flow and aids in the digestion of fats, reducing the risk of gallstone formation.

Regular Physical Activity:

Incorporating regular exercise into daily routines is key. Engaging in moderate physical activities like walking, jogging, or yoga not only helps in maintaining a healthy weight but also supports overall digestive health, reducing the likelihood of gallbladder issues linked to a sedentary lifestyle.

Stress Management and Relaxation Techniques:

Chronic stress can impact digestive health, including the gallbladder. Practicing stress-relieving techniques such as meditation, mindfulness, or deep breathing exercises helps in managing stress and its adverse effects on the digestive system.

Quality Sleep and Routine:

Establishing a consistent sleep schedule and ensuring adequate rest is crucial. Quality sleep supports overall well-being, including digestive health. Lack of proper sleep may contribute to increased stress levels, which can indirectly affect gallbladder function.

Avoidance of Harmful Habits:

Refraining from harmful habits like smoking, excessive alcohol consumption, and substance abuse is imperative. These habits can contribute to digestive issues and potentially exacerbate gallbladder problems.

Regular Check-ups and Monitoring:

Scheduled visits to healthcare professionals for routine check-ups and discussions about symptoms are essential. This proactive approach aids in early detection and prompt management of potential gallbladder concerns.

Conclusion:

Incorporating these lifestyle changes—maintaining hydration, regular physical activity, stress management, ensuring quality sleep, avoiding harmful habits, and regular medical check-ups—plays a pivotal role in supporting gallbladder function. By embracing these modifications, individuals adopt a proactive stance towards enhancing gallbladder health and promoting overall well-being. However, if we are to summarize, it can be said that the primary changes should indeed revolve around diet. Whether you like it or not, a problematic gallbladder will make you think twice before swallowing any morsel of food. Therefore, focus your main efforts on significant dietary changes and a balanced diet.

Physical Exercise: A Cornerstone of Gallbladder Health

While dietary modifications and stress management play crucial roles in maintaining gallbladder health, the importance of physical exercise cannot be overstated. Regular physical activity serves as a cornerstone in promoting overall well-being and specifically supports the intricate functions of the digestive system, including the gallbladder.

The Gallbladder-Exercise Connection:

At first glance, the link between exercise and gallbladder health might seem tenuous. However, delving deeper reveals a fascinating interplay between physical activity and this small yet vital organ. Exercise stimulates the contraction of the gallbladder, promoting the release of bile and preventing stagnation—a key factor in the formation of gallstones.

Moreover, regular physical activity aids in maintaining a healthy weight, reducing the risk of obesity-related gallbladder issues. It's a domino effect of wellness: as exercise helps manage weight, it indirectly supports gallbladder function by mitigating one of the primary risk factors for gallstone formation.

Tailored Exercises for Gallbladder Health:

1. **Walking: The Gentle Giant**. Don't underestimate the power of a brisk walk. This low-impact exercise, accessible to most individuals, stimulates digestion and promotes overall cardiovascular health. Aim for at least 30 minutes of walking daily, preferably after meals to aid in digestion and bile flow.

2. **Yoga: The Mind-Body Harmonizer**. Certain yoga poses can be particularly beneficial for gallbladder health. The "Bow Pose" (Dhanurasana) and "Twisted Chair Pose" (Parivrtta Utkatasana) gently massage the abdominal organs, potentially stimulating bile flow and aiding digestion. Always practice under the guidance of a qualified instructor, especially if you have existing gallbladder issues.

3. **Swimming: The Full-Body Elixir**. Swimming offers a full-body workout without putting undue stress on the joints. The rhythmic movements and controlled breathing involved in swimming can help reduce stress—a known contributor to digestive issues—while providing an excellent cardiovascular workout.

4. **Cycling: The Metabolic Booster**. Whether on a stationary bike or exploring outdoor trails, cycling is an excellent way to boost metabolism and support weight management. Start with shorter rides and gradually increase duration and intensity as your fitness improves.

5. **Resistance Training: Building Strength from Within.** Incorporating light to moderate resistance training into your routine can help maintain muscle mass and boost metabolism. Focus on compound exercises like squats, lunges, and push-ups, which engage multiple muscle groups simultaneously.

The Art of Moderation:

While exercise is undoubtedly beneficial, it's crucial to approach it with mindfulness, especially for those with existing gallbladder issues. High-intensity workouts or sudden, strenuous activities might trigger discomfort in some individuals. Listen to your body and gradually increase the intensity and duration of your workouts.

Hydration: The Often Overlooked Element

As you embark on your exercise journey, remember the importance of staying well-hydrated. Adequate water intake supports the body's natural detoxification processes and aids in maintaining the proper consistency of bile, reducing the risk of gallstone formation.

Consistency is Key:

The benefits of exercise for gallbladder health are cumulative. Consistency trumps intensity—regular, moderate exercise yields more sustainable benefits than sporadic, intense workouts. Aim to incorporate physical activity into your daily routine, making it as habitual as brushing your teeth.

A Holistic Approach:

Remember, exercise is just one piece of the puzzle in maintaining gallbladder health. Combine regular physical activity with a balanced diet, stress management techniques, and proper hydration for a comprehensive approach to gallbladder wellness.

Consultation is Crucial:

Before embarking on any new exercise regimen, especially if you have existing gallbladder issues or have undergone gallbladder surgery, consult with your healthcare provider. They can offer personalized advice and help tailor an exercise plan that aligns with your specific health needs and goals.

In conclusion, embracing regular physical activity is not just about sculpting your body or boosting cardiovascular health—it's a powerful tool in nurturing your gallbladder and overall digestive well-being. By incorporating these targeted exercises into your daily routine, you're taking a proactive step towards a healthier, more vibrant life, where your gallbladder functions optimally, supporting your body's intricate digestive processes.

Herbal and Alternative Remedies

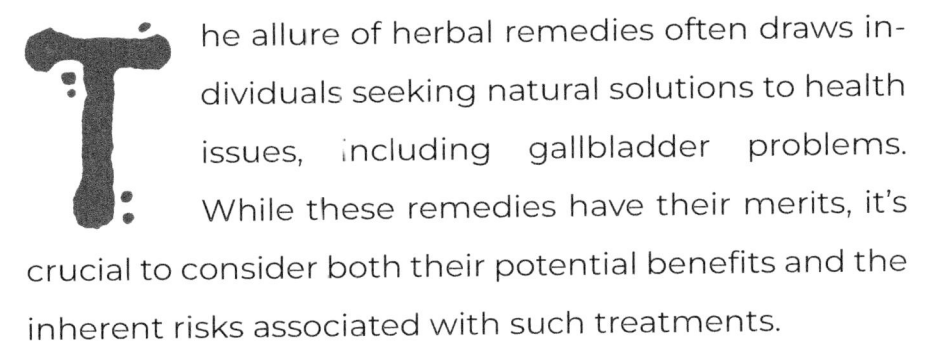

The allure of herbal remedies often draws individuals seeking natural solutions to health issues, including gallbladder problems. While these remedies have their merits, it's crucial to consider both their potential benefits and the inherent risks associated with such treatments.

The Lengthy Nature of Herbal Treatments:

Herbal treatments often necessitate a prolonged commitment. It can take years to observe significant improvements. However, this duration doesn't always guarantee sustained relief, especially in cases where the body is predisposed to gallstone formation. Despite investing considerable time in herbal treatments, recurrence remains a significant risk, creating a frustrating cycle.

Addressing Root Causes and Behavioral Patterns:

The crux of the matter lies beyond merely ingesting

herbal concoctions. It requires a shift in thinking and the management of emotions like anger and aggression. Failure to address these underlying issues can lead to a swift return of gallstones, undermining the efforts invested in herbal treatments.

The Perpetual Nature of Dietary Restrictions:

Moreover, herbal treatments often coincide with stringent dietary regimens. Even post-treatment, maintaining these dietary restrictions becomes a lifelong commitment. Are individuals prepared to embrace such a lifestyle, where dietary limitations persist as constant companions?

Herbs and Their Potential Benefits:

Certain herbs like milk thistle, dandelion root, and turmeric are believed to aid gallbladder health. Milk thistle supports liver function, potentially benefiting bile production. Dandelion root is thought to assist in bile flow. Turmeric, with its anti-inflammatory properties, might aid in alleviating gallbladder discomfort.

«Burdoch» or «burdock» (Arctium) is known for its medicinal properties and is sometimes used in traditional medicine to support digestive health. Its roots can be included in decoctions or infusions, believed to stimulate bile secretion and improve the overall functioning of the gallbladder. However, before using any herbs for medicinal purposes, it's important to consult with a healthcare professional, especially if there are any medical conditions or medications involved, to avoid potential negative interactions.

But there are numerous other herbs upon which healthcare professionals base their treatment systems, often confirming their effectiveness and appropriateness.

Conclusion:

While herbal remedies offer a natural approach to gallbladder issues, their efficacy is variable, and the commitment required extends beyond mere consumption. Addressing emotional triggers, maintaining restrictive diets, and the risk of recurrence demand considerable consideration. The decision to pursue herbal treatments should be made with a realistic understanding of their potential limitations and lifestyle adjustments they may necessitate. Consulting healthcare professionals is crucial for guidance tailored to individual needs and to weigh the benefits against the challenges of such alternative approaches.

Part II: Life After Gallbladder Removal

Understanding Cholecystectomy: Surgery and Recovery

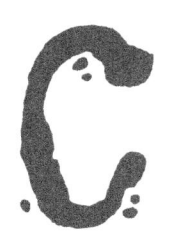

Cholecystectomy, the surgical removal of the gallbladder, stands as a crucial intervention for individuals grappling with gallstone-related issues or gallbladder inflammation. While the mere mention of surgery might induce anxiety, it's essential to understand the procedure's significance and its impact on one's life thereafter.

The gallbladder, though a part of the digestive system, is not indispensable for survival. Its primary function involves storing and concentrating bile produced by the liver. However, gallstones or inflammation can hinder its functionality, leading to severe abdominal pain, nausea, and other discomforting symptoms. In such cases, cholecystectomy becomes a viable solution.

The surgery itself can be performed through laparoscopic or open techniques. Laparoscopic procedures involve smaller incisions, resulting in quicker recovery times and minimal scarring, while open surgery necessitates a larger incision but might be required in more complex cases.

Post-surgery, patients may experience a brief hospital stay for observation. Recovery periods vary, but most individuals resume normal activities within a few weeks. Dietary adjustments might be recommended initially to accommodate changes in bile flow and aid in digestion.

Recovery after gallbladder removal surgery takes several months. The day after the operation, patients are advised to get up and move independently to prevent adhesions and stagnant processes. Wearing a special abdominal binder is also a mandatory requirement, significantly easing the recovery process. The binder should be worn for three months after the surgery.

Contrary to common belief, life after gallbladder removal often sees an improvement in quality. Relief from recurrent pain and discomfort linked to gallstones often leads to enhanced well-being. However, it's essential to dispel misconceptions about life without a gallbladder. While adaptation is necessary, many individuals lead fulfilling lives by making dietary adjustments and embracing healthy habits.

The fear associated with surgery should not overshadow its benefits. Cholecystectomy, while understandably daunting, is a routine and generally safe procedure. Complications are rare, and the benefits of alleviating gallbladder-related issues often outweigh the risks.

In conclusion, cholecystectomy signifies a resolution to persistent gallbladder issues. It represents an opportunity for improved health and relief from discomfort. Understanding the procedure, its implications, and focusing on post-surgery adjustments contribute to a smoother transition, allowing individuals to lead vibrant lives without the presence of their gallbladder.

Post-Surgery Diet and Nutrition

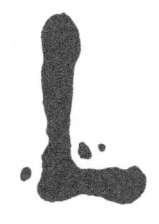

Laparoscopic gallbladder removal, or cholecystectomy, is considered minimally invasive, less traumatic surgery characterized by a quick recovery period and a low risk of complications.

The main condition for swift recovery and restoration of working capacity is the diet after laparoscopic cholecystectomy. Since the gallbladder, which served as a reservoir for bile and regulated its release into the duodenum, is absent, bile starts to discharge arbitrarily regardless of food intake. This can lead to several unpleasant complications such as cholecystitis, duodenitis, gastritis, colitis, and more.

Therefore, the post-cholecystectomy diet should heavily restrict products that stimulate bile until the bile ducts take over the function of the gallbladder and learn to partially accumulate bile.

Apart from restricting a list of products, the diet after laparoscopic cholecystectomy also involves a special feeding system—fractional eating. This means the patient should eat frequently but in small portions. Since, due to the absence of the gallbladder, bile has no place to accumulate, the quantity expelled through bile ducts might be insufficient to digest significant food portions.

The article further elaborates on the specifics of the post-cholecystectomy diet, the duration it needs to be followed, and provides an example of a healthy menu.

Post-Gallbladder Removal Diet during the Postoperative Period

As mentioned earlier, the diet following gallbladder removal via laparoscopy should be fractional. The patient should consume food 5-6 times a day in small portions. This type of eating after gallbladder removal (laparoscopy) ensures regular bile expulsion from the bile ducts, preventing bile stasis and the formation of stones.

The diet after gallbladder removal (laparoscopy) corresponds to diet table 195 according to Pevzner.

The prohibited list includes fatty meats and fish, concentrated broths, fried, spicy, salty, smoked, pickled, and canned products, fresh pastries, spinach, radishes, onions, garlic, legumes, chocolate, caviar, fresh fruits, carbonated drinks, coffee, strong tea, and alcoholic beverages. Vegetable oil intake is limited to 50 grams per day.

Allowed foods after cholecystectomy include lean meats and fish, light soups, lean broths, porridge, low-fat dairy products, stale bread, baked or lightly boiled fruits.

How Long to Follow the Diet after Gallbladder Removal

The diet after gallbladder removal (laparoscopy) should be followed until the bile ducts partially take on the function of the gallbladder and begin to accumulate and expel bile in necessary amounts for each meal.

Usually, the diet after gallbladder removal (cholecystectomy) is prescribed for at least six months.

For the initial 1.5-2 months after the surgery, it should be strict with maximum restriction of bile-stimulating products. Later, the menu can gradually expand, and for some patients, the diet after gallbladder removal (cholecystectomy) might be prescribed for a year or more.

Healthy Menu after Gallbladder Removal

Usually, a dietitian prepares a sample menu for the patient after gallbladder removal (laparoscopy). In the initial months, it should be strictly followed, and later, it can be slightly diversified.

CONCLUSION

In concluding this comprehensive guide, I extend my heartfelt gratitude to every reader who embarked on this journey toward gallbladder health and a fulfilling lifestyle. Together, we've navigated the intricate landscape of living without a gallbladder or striving to maintain its well-being.

My fervent hope is that this book has been more than just a guide; it's my aspiration that it has been a catalyst for positive change. For some, it may have provided solace, offering reassurance in making vital decisions about gallbladder health. To others, perhaps, it has alleviated the fear of living without this organ and shown that life can indeed be vibrant without it.

As an author deeply invested in the well-being of my readers, I sincerely hope that the insights shared within these pages have transformed lives for the better. Whether it's adopting healthier dietary habits, finding ways to manage pain, or embracing life after gallbladder removal, my aim was to empower and inspire.

Your decision to explore this guide demonstrates your commitment to your well-being, and for that, I am immensely grateful. I encourage you to embrace these newfound insights, integrate them into your daily life, and witness the positive changes they bring.

Wishing each of you continued success on your journey toward optimal health and well-being. May this book serve as a constant companion, offering guidance and support whenever needed.

Lastly, if this book has made a positive impact on your

life, I kindly invite you to share your experiences and leave a review on Amazon. Your feedback is invaluable, not only for me as an author but also for others seeking guidance on their path to gallbladder health.

Thank you for allowing me to be a part of your journey.

Warm regards

Literature

1. Townsend, C. M., Beauchamp, R. D., Evers, B. M., & Mattox, K. L. (2022). Sabiston Textbook of Surgery: The Biological Basis of Modern Surgical Practice. Elsevier.
2. Feldman, M., Friedman, L. S., & Brandt, L. J. (2020). Sleisenger and Fordtran's Gastrointestinal and Liver Disease. Elsevier.
3. Portincasa, P., Di Ciaula, A., de Bari, O., Garruti, G., Palmieri, V. O., & Wang, D. Q. H. (2016). Management of gallstones and its related complications. Expert Review of Gastroenterology & Hepatology, 10(1), 93-

112.

4. Stinton, L. M., & Shaffer, E. A. (2012). Epidemiology of gallbladder disease: cholelithiasis and cancer. Gut and liver, 6(2), 172.

5. Lammert, F., Gurusamy, K., Ko, C. W., Miquel, J. F., Méndez-Sánchez, N., Portincasa, P., ... & Wang, D. Q. H. (2016). Gallstones. Nature Reviews Disease Primers, 2(1), 1-17.

6. Kwo, P. Y., Cohen, S. M., & Lim, J. K. (2017). ACG Clinical Guideline: Evaluation of Abnormal Liver Chemistries. American Journal of Gastroenterology, 112(1), 18-35.

7. Bouchier, I. A. D., & Freston, J. W. (2019). The Oxford Textbook of Clinical Hepatology. Oxford University Press.

8. European Association for the Study of the Liver (EASL). (2016). EASL Clinical Practice Guidelines on the prevention, diagnosis and treatment of gallstones. Journal of Hepatology, 65(1), 146-181.

Printed in Great Britain
by Amazon